ESSENTIAL GUIDE TO LIPOMA

Comprehensive Insights into Lipoma Management and Care

DR. CASEY LOREN

DISCLAIMER

This book's content is only meant to be used for general informative purposes. Although the author has taken great care to ensure the content is accurate and thorough, no warranties or assurances on the information's accuracy, correctness, or reliability are provided. It is recommended that readers employ their own judgment and discretion when applying any material found in this book to their particular situation.

The information in this book is not intended to replace professional advice, nor is the author an expert in any of the subjects covered. It is recommended that readers consult with experienced professionals regarding any particular issues or concerns.

Any name that may be mentioned or referred in this book does not imply endorsement, recommendation, or relationship on the part of the author with any person, entity, good, website, or association. These references are made only for informational purposes and are not meant to be taken as recommendations or endorsements.

The information contained in this book may cause readers to suffer loss or damage, for which the author disclaims all obligation and accountability. The only people accountable for the decisions and actions taken by readers using the information presented are themselves.

Any names, characters, companies, locations, activities, occasions, and incidents referenced in this book are either made up or the result of the author's imagination. Any likeness to real people, living or dead, or to real things is entirely coincidental.

This book's content may change at any time, without prior notice, according to the author. The onus is on the reader to verify whether there have been any updates or revisions.

The reader accepts the conditions of this disclaimer by reading this book. Please do not read this book or use its contents if you do not agree to these terms.

Table of Contents

CHAPTER 1

COMPREHENDING LIPOMA

Lipoma Definition

A lipoma is a type of benign tumor made up of fat cells called adipose tissue. Usually, it feels like a rubbery, squishy lump beneath the skin that moves readily when applied with light pressure. Lipomas can develop in any place in the body where there are fat cells, and they often cause little pain as they grow slowly. Although lipomas are normally benign, they can occasionally cause pain or aesthetic problems, prompting people to seek medical attention for diagnosis and treatment.

Lipoma Types

Based on their characteristics and location, lipomas can be classified into numerous types:

1. The most prevalent kind, called superficial subcutaneous lipomatosis, is found immediately below the skin's surface.

2. Lipomas profundas intramusculares: These form inside the muscles.

3. Lipoma intermusculare: These lipomas develop in between muscles.

4. Intradermal Lipomas: These types of lipomas are located deep within the skin's layers.

Lipoma Causes

Although the precise cause of lipomas is unknown, several variables may be involved in their development:

1. hereditary Factors: There may be a hereditary susceptibility to lipomas since they can run in families.

2. Hormonal Factors: Variations in hormone levels, including those that occur during pregnancy, may have an impact on the development of lipomas.

3. Trauma: Lesions or trauma to regions of fatty tissue may occasionally result in the development of lipomas.

4. Obesity: Although it is not a direct cause, obesity may make lipomas more likely to develop.

Lipoma symptoms

Typical signs and symptoms of lipomas include:

1. a doughy, mushy lump beneath the skin.

2. The lump is easily moved with light pressure.

3. Though some people may feel tenderness or discomfort, it is usually painless.

4. gradual expansion in magnitude over time.

5. seldom linked to systemic symptoms like fever or loss of weight.

Lipoma diagnosis

Identifying a lipoma usually entails:

1. Physical Examination: The size, texture, and mobility of the lump will be evaluated by a medical professional.

2. Imaging Tests: To see the location and features of the lipoma, an MRI or ultrasound scan may be performed.

3. Biopsy: To confirm the diagnosis and rule out other illnesses, a biopsy may occasionally be carried out.

The following are risk factors for lipomatosis:

The following variables may make developing lipomas more likely:

1. Family History: The risk of acquiring lipomas is increased if a family member already has one.

2. Age: Middle-aged adults are more likely to have lipomas.

3. Gender: Males are slightly more likely than females to have lipomas.

4. Genetic abnormalities: An increased risk of lipoma formation is linked to certain genetic abnormalities.

What Distinguishes Lipoma from Liposarcoma?

Despite including adipose tissue, lipomas and liposarcomas differ greatly in terms of malignancy:

1. Lipoma: A benign tumor that grows slowly and is rarely invasive, consisting of mature fat cells.

2. Liposarcoma: A malignant tumor that originates from fat cells, grows quickly, and can spread to neighboring tissues.

Lipoma Incidence and Prevalence

According to estimates, lipomas affect roughly 1% of the population. They are a prevalent condition. Although they can happen at any age, adults between the ages of 40 and 60 are the ones who are diagnosed with them the most often. People with specific genetic disorders or a family history of lipomas are more likely to develop lipomas.

Lipoma Across Various Age Groups

Although lipomas can develop at any age, their prevalence varies depending on the age group:

1. Children and Adolescents: Although lipomas are uncommon in this age range, they can nevertheless happen, frequently in single cases or as part of hereditary disorders.

2. Adults: Adults, especially those in their middle years, are the ones who get lipomas diagnosed the most frequently.

3. Elderly: Although they might not occur as frequently as in younger age groups, lipomas can nevertheless form in senior persons.

Recent Studies on Lipoma

The following areas are the focus of ongoing research on lipomas:

1. Genetic Studies: Examining the hereditary components that underlie the formation and inheritance patterns of lipomas.

2. Molecular biology: Knowing the molecular pathways that promote the growth of lipomas and possible targets for treatment.

3. Imaging Techniques: Improving the identification and diagnosis of lipomas through the development of imaging technology.

4. Treatment Modalities: Investigating cutting-edge approaches to effectively manage lipomas, such as targeted medicines or less invasive procedures.

This in-depth manual attempts to give readers a complete grasp of lipomas by going over their definitions, types, causes, symptoms, diagnosis, risk factors, prevalence in various age groups, and current research initiatives.

CHAPTER 3

PHYSIOLOGY AND ANATOMY

Structure of Adipose Tissue

Often referred to as fat tissue, adipocytes, or fat cells, make up the majority of the specialized connective tissue known as adipose tissue. Triglycerides, which are energy-storing lipid droplets, are present throughout these cells. There are two primary forms of adipose tissue: brown adipose tissue (BAT) and white adipose tissue (WAT). While BAT is engaged in thermogenesis, which produces heat, WAT stores energy and cushions organs.

Adipose Tissue Functions

1. **Energy Storage:** Triglycerides, which are extra energy, are stored by adipose tissue and released as needed for metabolic functions.

2. **Insulation:** Adipose tissue beneath the skin acts as thermal insulation to control body temperature.

3. Adipose tissue shields internal organs from mechanical shocks by providing cushioning.

4. **Endocrine Function:** Hormones (adipokines) secreted by adipose tissue control hunger, inflammation, and metabolism.

Process of Lipoma Formation

A lipoma is a type of benign adipose tissue tumor. The process of formation entails:

1. **Proliferation:** An excessive number of adipocytes proliferate to create a bulk of fat tissue.

2. **Encapsulation:** A fibrous capsule encloses the bulk and isolates it from the surrounding tissues.

3. **Growth:** Lipomas can vary in size from a few millimeters to several centimeters, and they can grow slowly over time.

Elements Influencing Lipoma Development

The following variables may affect how lipomas grow:

1. **Genetics:** There may be a hereditary predisposition to lipomas since they can run in families.

2. **Obesity:** The development of lipomas may be facilitated by an increase in adipose tissue in obese people.

3. **Hormonal Changes:** Adipose tissue growth may be impacted by hormonal imbalances or modifications.

4. **Age:** Although they can happen at any age, lipomas are more common in middle-aged individuals.

5. **Trauma:** Adipose tissue trauma or damage may be the cause of lipoma development.

Lipoma Sites in the Human Body

Lipomas can develop anywhere on the body, including:

1. **Subcutaneous:** Under the skin, usually on the arms, thighs, neck, and trunk.

2. **Intramuscular:** Inside muscles; frequently seen during scans or operations.

3. **Visceral:** Inside internal organs including the kidneys, liver, or gastrointestinal tract (rare).

Lipoma's Effect on Adjacent Tissues

Although lipomas are usually benign, they can put pressure on the tissues around them, which might result in:

1. **Discomfort:** If large lipomas squeeze blood vessels or nerves, they may be painful or uncomfortable.

2. **Cosmetic problems:** Visible lipomas may give rise to cosmetic problems.

3. **Functional Impairment:** Certain lipomas can cause problems with organ function or movement.

Growth Patterns of Lipomas

Lipomas can grow in a variety of ways:

1. **Slow Growth:** Over months or years, most lipomas grow slowly.

2. **Stable Size:** Some lipomas don't significantly alter in size over time.

3. **Rapid Growth:** Rarely, lipomas may grow quickly, necessitating evaluation and medical intervention.

Variability in Lipomas' Size

The size of lipomas can range from tiny nodules to massive masses. Variability in size is dependent upon things like:

1. **Duration:** Longer lipomas typically have a bigger diameter.

2. **Location:** Lipomas in specific regions, like the thighs or back, may enlarge before being discovered.

3. **Individual Variation:** While some people may have fewer, larger lipomas, others may develop several little ones.

Lipoma Structure

The components of a lipoma consist of:

1. **Adipocytes:** Mostly made up of mature fat cells with lots of lipid droplets, or adipocytes.

2. **Fibrous Capsule:** Fibrous connective tissue encapsulates lipomas.

3. ** Blood Supply:** Compared to malignant tumors, lipomas have a smaller blood supply.

Problems with Lipomas

Although lipomas are typically benign, they can cause issues like:

1. **Discomfort:** More substantial lipomas or those putting pressure on nerves may be painful.

2. **Cosmetic Concerns:** Self-image may be impacted by lipomas in conspicuous regions.

3. **Functional Impairment:** Lipomas close to organs or joints may cause problems with function or mobility.

4. **Diagnostic Challenges:** Imaging or biopsy may be necessary to differentiate lipomas from malignant tumors.

CHAPTER 3

LIPOMA DIAGNOSIS

Lipoma Physical Examination

A complete examination and palpation of the afflicted area are usually part of a physical evaluation for lipoma. Under the skin, lipomas frequently appear as moveable, squishy lumps that are rubbery. They often grow gradually and without pain. In addition to evaluating the lipoma's dimensions, location, texture, and shape, the examiner may also ask about any accompanying symptoms, such as discomfort or size fluctuations.

Imaging Methods for the Diagnosis of Lipomas:

Imaging is essential for the diagnosis of lipomas. Ultrasound, magnetic resonance imaging (MRI), and computed tomography (CT) scans are examples of common methods. Since ultrasound is inexpensive and can distinguish between lipomas and other soft tissue tumors, it is frequently utilized as a first-line imaging technique. MRI offers high-resolution pictures and is especially helpful in determining the extent of a lipoma and how it interacts with adjacent structures. When accurate anatomical localization is necessary, CT scans may be used.

Lipoma Biopsy Procedures:

Although imaging results and clinical examinations are usually sufficient to diagnose lipomas, a biopsy may be necessary in some circumstances to confirm the diagnosis or rule out other illnesses. Core needle biopsy or fine-needle aspiration (FNA) biopsy may be used; FNA is a less invasive method. It's crucial to remember that a biopsy is typically saved for unusual or questionable instances and is not always required for the diagnosis of lipoma.

Differential Lipoma Diagnosis:

Because lipomas can resemble other soft tissue tumors, it's critical to make a differential diagnosis. Considerable conditions include benign tumors of various tissues, neurofibromas, sebaceous cysts, epidermoid cysts, and liposarcoma, a malignant tumor of fat cells. The differentiation of these entities is aided by clinical assessment, imaging investigations, and occasionally biopsy.

Difficulties in Diagnosing Lipomas:

Although the diagnosis of lipomas is usually simple, unusual cases like deep-seated or intra-abdominal lipomas can present difficulties. In many cases, precise diagnosis and treatment planning depend on imaging methods and potentially biopsies.

Systems of Lipoma Grading:

Unlike malignant tumors, lipomas are usually benign and do not have a grading system. On the other hand, other classification schemes—like superficial vs deep-seated lipomas or infiltrative versus non-infiltrative variations—are predicated on histological characteristics. Treatment choices may be influenced by this categorization.

Lipoma Surveillance and Aftercare:

Most lipomas are benign and asymptomatic once they are discovered, therefore no quick action is necessary. Nonetheless, it could be advised to follow up and examine the patient regularly to record any changes in size, symptoms, or appearance. This is especially crucial when the lipoma is big, expanding quickly, or causing pain.

Recurrence Rates of Lipomas:

Lipomas are renowned for having low rates of recurrence following surgical excision. Recurrence, however, is possible, particularly if the lipoma is not completely removed after surgery. Recurrence risk may be raised by elements like inadequate resection or the existence of numerous lipomas.

Cases of Lipomatosis Misdiagnosis:

Misdiagnosis of lipomas can happen, resulting in unwarranted worry or unsuitable interventions. Sebaceous cysts, epidermoid cysts, neurofibromas, and liposarcomas are among the common misdiagnoses. Misinterpretation can be prevented by clinical correlation, imaging investigations, and even biopsy.

Innovations in Lipoma Diagnosis:

The diagnosis of lipomas is becoming more accurate thanks to developments in imaging technology including high-resolution ultrasonography and magnetic resonance imaging. Furthermore, genomic and genetic investigations may provide information on the pathophysiology of lipomas and help differentiate between benign and malignant lesions.

CHAPTER 4

OPTIONS FOR TREATMENT

Alternative Medicine for Lipoma:

Steroid injections, lipolysis, and observation are non-surgical therapy options for lipomas. Observation entails keeping an eye out for modifications to the lipoma's size, shape, or symptoms. Injections of steroids can be used to shrink the size and reduce inflammation, but they are not always successful. Lipolysis is the process of injecting a material into the lipoma to break down the fat cells.

Techniques for Surgical Removal:

Excision is the usual method used in surgery to remove lipomas; the surgeon makes an incision, removes the lipoma, and sutures the wound up. For smaller lipomas, smaller incisions are made when using minimal excision techniques. Endoscopic removal removes the lipoma by inserting tiny equipment and a camera through tiny incisions.

Benefits and Risks of Surgery for Lipomatosis:

Lipoma surgery carries several hazards, including bleeding, infection, scarring, nerve injury, and recurrence. Nonetheless, lipomas that cause pain, discomfort, or cosmetic issues can frequently be removed surgically. Improvements in look and symptom reduction are among the advantages.

After Surgery Recuperation:

The location, size, and surgical method of a lipoma all affect how well a patient recovers from the procedure. At first, patients may have discomfort, bruising, edema, and limited movement. Throughout their recuperation period, which can last anywhere from a few days to several weeks, patients should adhere to the post-operative care guidelines.

Lipoma Excision in Various Body Parts:

re several body parts where lipomas can develop, such as the arms, legs, trunk, neck, and head. Depending on the location and size of the lipoma, different surgical techniques may be used. For instance, more careful surgical methods could be needed for lipomas in delicate regions like the face or neck.

Liposuction to Remove a Lipoma:

In some circumstances, lipoma removal may be accomplished with liposuction, especially for big or many lipomas. With this method, the fatty tissue surrounding the lipoma is suctioned out using a thin tube called a cannula. While less intrusive than standard surgery, liposuction might not be an appropriate treatment for every lipoma.

Lipoma and Cryolipolysis:

Known colloquially as "fat freezing," cryolipolysis is a non-surgical technique that employs low temperatures to kill fat cells. Although it has been used to reduce fat cosmetically, research is still needed to determine how successful it is in treating lipomas, therefore it might not be highly advised.

Treatment with Radiation for Lipoma:

Because there is little chance that lipomas can develop into cancer, radiation therapy is rarely utilized to treat lipomas.

But in some situations where surgery is not practical or efficient, it might be taken into consideration. High-energy beams are used in radiation therapy to target and reduce the lipoma.

Lipoma Alternative Therapies:

Acupuncture, homeopathy, and herbal medicines are examples of alternative therapies for lipoma. Nevertheless, there isn't much scientific data to back up their efficacy in treating lipomas. It's crucial to speak with a medical expert before attempting any alternative treatments.

Potential Directions for Lipoma Therapy:

The treatment of lipomas may evolve in the future to include non-surgical methods such as focused ultrasound, laser therapy, or targeted medication therapies. Research is being done to create less invasive and more accurate ways to identify and treat lipomas.

CHAPTER 5

COEXISTING WITH LIPOMA

Lipoma's Psychological Effects

People who have lipoma may experience psychological effects. Feelings of self-consciousness could result from it, particularly if the lipoma is noticeable and has an impact on appearance. Some people may go through periods of anxiety or despair because they worry about the lipoma spreading or about how other people will see them. People must talk about these emotions and get help when they need it.

Lipoma Patients' Coping Techniques

Lipoma patients have several coping mechanisms at their disposal to assist them cope with their illness. These include learning as much as you can about lipoma, being honest and upfront with medical professionals, engaging in stress-relieving techniques like mindfulness or meditation, asking friends and family for support, and concentrating on interests and pursuits that make you happy and fulfilled.

Resources and Support Groups

Patients with lipomas may find information and support groups to be beneficial. These groups give people a place to connect with people who can relate to their experiences, exchange knowledge and advice, and provide emotional support. Resources such as social media groups, local support groups run by healthcare organizations, and online forums can be very beneficial.

Modifications to Lifestyle for the Management of Lipoma

Although lifestyle changes are not a cure for lipoma, they can help control symptoms and enhance general health. This could entail exercising frequently, controlling stress levels, eating a balanced diet, abstaining from smoking, and consuming little or no alcohol.

Physical Activity and Lipomas

For patients with lipomas, frequent physical exercise can be helpful. Exercise can enhance mood, lower stress levels, increase circulation, and support general health. Before beginning any new fitness program, people should speak with their doctor, especially if they have large or painful lipomas.

Dietary Considerations for Lipomas

Although there isn't a particular diet for lipoma management, following a healthy, balanced diet helps improve general health. Consuming an abundance of fruits, vegetables, whole grains, lean meats, and healthy fats is part of this. Some people may decide to restrict or stay away from foods that are heavy in processed carbohydrates, harmful fats, or sugar.

Interactions with Lipoma

Relationships may be impacted by lipomatosis, especially if the condition makes a person feel uncomfortable or self-conscious. Maintaining open lines of communication about lipoma and its effects with friends, family, and partners helps provide understanding and support.

Lipoma and Work

The majority of people with lipomas can work normally. Nonetheless, adjustments at work can be required if the lipoma results in pain, discomfort, or restricted mobility. This could involve changing the duties, being flexible with the schedule, or making ergonomic improvements. To guarantee a supportive work environment, individuals must maintain communication with their employer and healthcare practitioner.

Lipoma in Juveniles and Teens

Lipoma is less prevalent in children and adolescents than in adults, although it can still happen. Unless they cause pain or other symptoms, lipomas in this age group are usually benign and don't need to be treated. If parents observe any strange lumps or changes in their child's health, they should get in touch with a healthcare expert.

Quality of Life and Lipomas:

The effects of lipomas on an individual's quality of life vary based on several factors, including size, location, symptoms, and personal experiences. Lipomas are generally benign and don't significantly interfere with day-to-day activities. However, quality of life may be compromised for certain people, particularly for those with bigger or symptomatic lipomas. Patients must collaborate with medical professionals to manage their symptoms and take care of any quality-of-life issues.

CHAPTER 6

MYTHS AND FACTS ABOUT LIPOMAS

The Ultimate Lipoma Guide: Myths and Reality

Frequently Held Myths Regarding Lipomas

Benign tumors made of fat tissue are called lipomas. There are still a few prevalent myths, though:

- **Myth: Cancerous lipomas exist.**

Fact: Lipomas do not cause cancer and are benign. They don't spread to other tissues or invade them; they are made up of fully developed fat cells.

Illogical belief: Lipomas invariably enlarge.

Fact: Over time, many lipomas don't change in size; however, others may increase. Fast growth is unusual and needs to be assessed by a medical specialist.

Illogical belief: Diet and exercise alone can eradicate lipomas.

Fact: Losing weight or altering one's lifestyle does not affect lipomas. To remove them, medical or surgical intervention is necessary.

Myth: People who are overweight are the only ones who get lipomas.

Fact: People with lipomas can have any sort of body. There is a greater influence from genetics and other elements.

Home Remedies for Lipoma

Numerous traditional medicines have been proposed for the treatment of lipomas throughout history:

- **Herbal Remedies:** Some people think that using herbs like chickweed, flaxseed oil, and turmeric will help lower the size of lipomas. Nevertheless, these assertions are unsupported by any scientific data.

- **Apple Cider Vinegar:** Thought to decrease lipomas, apple cider vinegar is a popular home remedy that lacks scientific support.

Essential Oils: Although there is no clinical evidence to support the effectiveness of oils like frankincense and tea tree oil in treating lipomas, they are occasionally advised.

Even while these treatments are usually safe, they shouldn't be used in place of expert medical guidance or care.

Busting Myths About Lipomas

Myths about lipomas can cause unwarranted anxiety and confusion.

Myth: Cancer can develop from lipomas.

Reality: Lipomas do not progress to malignancy and are benign. A distinct, unrelated type of cancer is called liposarcoma, which is an uncommon illness.

Myth: Trauma or injury is the cause of lipomas.

Truth: There is no proof that physical trauma causes lipomas to occur. Genetic factors are most likely the cause of them.

- **Myth: There is a spread of lipomas.**

Fact: There is no way for lipomas to spread from one person to another. They do not spread illness.

Misconceptions Regarding Lipoma and Cancer

Many times, people misunderstand the connection between lipomas and cancer.

To be clear, lipomas are benign tumors. They don't make getting cancer more likely.

- **Concern:** To rule out other disorders, any quick changes in a lipoma, such as sudden growth or pain, should be evaluated by a physician.

- **Differentiation:** Lipomas are different from liposarcomas, a kind of malignancy. An appropriate medical examination can distinguish between the two.

The Social Shame Around Lipomas

People with lipomas may face social stigma:

- **Body Image:** Visible lipomas may result in social disengagement or anxiety due to feelings of humiliation or self-consciousness.

- **Misunderstanding:** People may judge or show misplaced worry if they are unaware of lipomas.

Support: Promoting understanding and lowering stigma can be achieved by fostering candid conversation and disseminating correct information.

Popular Culture's Use of Lipoma

Sometimes seen in popular culture, lipomas are frequently misinterpreted.

- **Media Depiction:** Lipomas may be portrayed falsely in films and television programs, which may exaggerate their consequences or make them appear more serious than they are.

* **Impact:** These depictions have the potential to spread false beliefs and prejudices, influencing public opinion.

Well-Known Persons with Lipoma

Numerous well-known people have experienced lipomas:

- **As an illustration, consider the late Steve Jobs, a co-founder of Apple, who misdiagnosed a lipoma as a more serious illness.

- **Influence:** Sharing personal accounts from well-known people with lipomas might help dispel stigma and demystify the illness.

Lipoma's Media Representation

Public perception is significantly shaped by media representation:

Accuracy: To prevent false information from spreading, media representations of lipomas must be factual.

- **Awareness:** Accurate and uplifting media coverage helps inform the public and promote compassion for individuals afflicted with the illness.

Effect of False Information on Lipomas

False information regarding lipomas can have several detrimental effects:

- **Health Decisions:** Uninformed people can put off getting medical advice or choose ineffective over-the-counter treatments.

- **Emotional Stress:** Having misconceptions about lipomas might lead to unwarranted dread and anxiety.

- **Public Perception:** Misconceptions that are widely held can reinforce stigma and misunderstanding.

Teaching People About Lipomas

Fighting stigma and misinformation around lipomas requires education:

- **Accurate Information:** Provide scientific information and credible references regarding lipomas.

- **Personal Narratives:** To humanize lipomas, invite people who have them to relate their stories.

Expert Advice: Stress the significance of seeking medical advice from professionals for diagnosis and treatment.

CHAPTER 7

MEDICAL RESEARCH AND LIPOMAS

Essential Lipoma Guide: All-Inclusive Views

Studies on Lipoma Pathogenesis

Mature adipocytes form benign tumors known as lipomas. Numerous processes, such as dysregulated cell signaling pathways, genetic abnormalities, and local trauma, contribute to the pathophysiology of lipomas. The function of the HMGA2 gene, which codes for a protein essential in controlling cell growth and differentiation, has been brought to light by research. In lipoma cells, aberrant expression or rearrangement of HMGA2 has been often seen. Furthermore, research indicates that mild traumas or local stress may cause lipoma production by inducing an inflammatory response that accelerates the growth of adipocytes.

Variables in the Development of Lipomas

The formation of lipomas is significantly influenced by genetic predisposition. Multiple lipomas within families are indicative of a hereditary component in the illness known as familial multiple lipomatosis. Lipomas have been linked to specific genetic changes, including rearrangements of the 12q13–15 and 6p21–23 chromosomal regions. The pathophysiology of lipoma has been linked to mutations in the MEN1 gene, which is linked to multiple endocrine neoplasia type 1, and the HMGA2 gene. Knowing these genetic variables aids in risk assessment and could direct future treatment approaches.

Lipoma Immunohistochemical Markers

A useful technique for identifying lipomas and distinguishing them from other soft tissue tumors is immunohistochemistry (IHC). S-100 protein is a common IHC marker for lipoma and is frequently positive in adipocytes. Atypical lipomatous tumors, or well-differentiated liposarcomas, are malignant tumors that may be distinguished from lipomas using markers like MDM2 and CDK4. These indicators' expression aids pathologists in correctly diagnosing lipomas and ensuring the best possible clinical care.

Research on Lipoma and Adipose Tissue

Studying lipomas reveals information on the biology of adipose tissue. In addition to serving as a store of energy, adipose tissue is an endocrine organ that controls metabolism. Research on lipomas, which are aberrant adipose tissue formations, can provide light on lipid metabolism, adipogenesis, and the function of adipokines, or fat cell-secreted hormones, in both health and sickness. The findings of this study have significance for our knowledge of metabolic diseases, obesity, and possible treatment targets.

Projects to Map the Lipoma Genome

The goal of genome mapping initiatives is to locate genetic alterations and variants linked to the emergence of lipomas. Through the sequencing of lipoma tissue genomes, scientists can identify particular genetic mutations and processes that contribute to the development of tumors. To find recurring mutations and gene rearrangements, these initiatives frequently use bioinformatics analysis and next-generation sequencing technology. The information gathered may help identify new therapy targets and individualized care plans.

Lipoma Research Using Animal Models

To better understand lipoma biology and evaluate possible therapies, animal models are crucial. Transgenic mice carrying mutations in genes such as MEN1 or HMGA2 can develop tumors resembling lipomas, which makes them useful as models for researching the genesis and spread of tumors. Before human clinical trials, these models enable researchers to examine the genetic and cellular pathways underlying the creation of lipomas and assess the safety and effectiveness of novel therapy strategies.

Lipoma Medication Research

The goal of lipoma drug development is to identify non-surgical ways to shrink or remove tumors. The application of lipolytic drugs, which degrade fat cells, and inhibitors of particular signaling pathways implicated in the growth of adipocytes is being investigated in current research. For example, medications that target the PI3K/AKT/mTOR pathway—which is frequently dysregulated in lipomas—are being researched. If a patient has several or recurring lipomas, effective medication therapy may offer an option for surgical removal.

Clinical Trials for Treatments of Lipomatosis

Clinical studies are essential for assessing novel lipoma therapies. These studies evaluate the effectiveness and safety of cutting-edge medications, minimally invasive treatments, and innovative surgical methods. Recent studies have looked into treating lipomas with injectable deoxycholic acid, a fat-dissolving agent. Gene therapy and targeted molecular therapies are the subjects of other research. Clinical trial participation advances medical knowledge while providing patients with access to cutting-edge treatments.

Funding for Lipoma Research

Funding for lipoma research is crucial to improving our understanding of the disease and creating novel therapies. Governmental organizations, private foundations, and pharmaceutical firms are some of the funding sources. Basic and clinical research projects are supported by grants from organizations such as the European Research Council (ERC) and the National Institutes of Health (NIH). Funding for research projects also heavily depends on cooperation between academics, businesses, and patient advocacy organizations.

Joint Ventures in Lipoma Studies

The breadth and significance of lipoma research are increased when scientists, physicians, and organizations work together. Complex research topics can be addressed by multidisciplinary teams that combine skills in pathology, genetics, molecular biology, and clinical medicine. Large-scale investigations and data sharing are made easier by international consortia and research networks, which speeds up discovery.

CHAPTER 8

CASE STUDIES

Difficulties in Diagnosing Lipomatosis

The diagnosis of lipomatosis might be difficult since it resembles other soft tissue lumps. Patients frequently arrive with a soft, moveable, painless lump beneath the skin. For appropriate therapy, it is imperative to differentiate a lipoma from other medical disorders such as liposarcoma, cysts, or fib

- **Limited Scope of Clinical Examination**: A physical examination may not be able to definitively distinguish lipomas from malignant tumors.

- **Imaging Techniques**: CT, MRI, and ultrasound scans are helpful, but the results can still be unclear.

- **Biopsy Considerations**: Although excisional biopsy or fine needle aspiration can confirm the diagnosis, there is a chance of complications or sample mistakes.

- **Unusual Presentations**: Rapid growth is one unusual aspect of some lipomas that raises the possibility of malignancy.

Effective Treatment for Lipomas

Surgical removal is usually required for successful treatment of lipomas; depending on the size and location of the lipoma, this procedure can be simple or complex. Important details consist of:

- **Surgical Techniques**: Less invasive methods, liposuction-assisted removal, and straightforward excision are available.

Preoperative Planning: To reduce risks and guarantee total excision, precise imaging and thorough planning are necessary.

Postoperative Care: This involves dressing wounds, keeping an eye out for infections, and making sure healing is adequate to stop recurrence.

- **Patient Satisfaction**: The degree to which the patient is satisfied with the cosmetic result and the absence of any symptoms is another way to gauge success.

Management of Lipoma Recurrence

Lipomas can recur and this can be troublesome. Controlling recurrences entails:

- **Determining Recurrence Causes**: Recurrences may arise from incomplete removal, multiple lipomas, or hereditary susceptibility (such as in familial multiple lipomatosis).

- **Reoperation Strategies**: Carefully excising recurrent lipomas while keeping in mind the locations of prior surgeries.

Follow-Up Protocols: Imaging studies and routine follow-up visits to check for new growths.

- **Patient Education**: Educating patients on recurrence warning signals and urging prompt medical attention if they develop new lumps.

Lipoma in Unusual Places

Unusual sites for lipomas can present special complications.

- **Intramuscular Lipomas**: Pain and functional impairment may result from these masses, which are located within muscles.

Rare and capable of mimicking other intra-abdominal masses are **Intra-abdominal Lipomas**.

- **Spinal Cord Lipomas**: These conditions can cause neurological symptoms and necessitate intricate surgical procedures.

- **Diagnosis and Treatment**: For lipomas in unusual places, specialized imaging and surgical experience are frequently required.

Paediatric Patients with Lipomas

Although less prevalent in children, lipomas require special precautions.

- **Diagnostic Approach**: Making sure a benign lipoma is not misdiagnosed as a pediatric tumor of more concern.

- **Growth Monitoring**: Since children are still developing, it is crucial to regularly examine the lipoma's growth and how it affects the surrounding tissues.

Surgical Intervention: When it comes to anesthesia and postoperative care, pediatric patients need to be given extra attention.

Coexisting Conditions and Lipoma

Management of lipomas can be complicated when they coincide with other medical conditions:

Diabetes: Poor wound healing following surgery and an increased risk of infection.

Obesity: Increased risk of recurrent lipomas and problems following surgery.

- **Genetic Conditions**: These include several lipomas and the need for a more comprehensive approach to treatment, such as Madelung's disease or familial multiple lipomatosis.

- **Management Strategies**: Effective coexisting condition management involves coordinated care with various specialists.

Elderly Patients' Lipoma

When treating lipomas in older people, particular considerations must be made:

Age-Related Risks: Surgical risks associated with comorbid conditions such as diabetes or heart disease are higher.

- **Fragile Skin**: Slower healing and a higher risk of skin problems.

- **Non-Surgical Options**: These include observation or less intrusive treatments; sometimes chosen due to lesser risk.

- **Quality of Life**: Prioritise preserving functionality and reducing discomfort.

Psychological Effects of Lipoma

Lipomas can have a major psychological impact:

- **Body Image Issues**: Self-consciousness and negative body image might result from visible or big lipomas.

Anxiety: Worries about the lump's nature and possible cancerous nature.

- **Supportive Care**: Reducing anxiety can be achieved by offering psychological support, counseling, and unambiguous information regarding the benign nature of the illness.

Case Study 9: Complications with Lipomas

Preface

Lipomas are slow-growing, mostly benign tumors made of fat cells. Even though they are usually benign, there may be some difficulties, especially if the lipoma grows to a large size or under uncommon conditions.

Typical Lipoma Complications

1. **Agony and Unease**

Compression of Nerves: More substantial lipomas may put pressure on adjacent nerves, resulting in pain or discomfort.

- **Muscle Interference**: Lipomas may occasionally cause problems with the function or movement of muscles, particularly if they are located in a region that moves often.

2. **Contagious**

- **Surface Infection**: A lipoma may get infected, even though it is uncommon, especially if it is hurt or becomes ulcerated. Warmth, soreness, and redness are some of the symptoms.

- **Abscess Formation**: Drainage and antibiotics may be necessary if an infected lipoma turns into an abscess.

3. **Inflammation**

- **Lipomatosis**: When there are several lipomas, there may be extensive inflammation, which can result in systemic symptoms including fever and malaise.

4. **Scald**

- **Skin Ulceration**: Because of pressure and decreased blood flow to the skin above, large or subcutaneous lipomas can occasionally result in skin ulcers.

5. **Disruption to Organ Performance**

- **Intramuscular Lipomas**: These lipomas can develop inside muscle tissue, resulting in discomfort and perhaps impairing muscle function.

- **Visceral Lipomas**: In rare cases, lipomas can form in or close to internal organs, which can cause problems if they are in the gastrointestinal system. One such problem is bowel blockage.

Misdiagnosis of Lipomas

Preface

Misdiagnosis can happen even though lipomas are usually simple to diagnose with clinical examination and imaging. Misdiagnosis might cause more dangerous illnesses that mirror lipomas to go unnoticed or result in needless therapies.

Frequently Occurring Disorders Mislabeled as Lipomas

1. **Tumours Lipomatous**

- **Liposarcoma**: An aggressive malignant fatty tissue tumor that requires a different course of treatment than a lipoma.

- **Angiolipoma**: Unlike other lipomas, this one has vascular components and may cause pain when it first appears.

2. **Conditions Not Lipomatous**

Fibroma: A benign fibrous tissue tumor with a similar appearance to a lipoma that can be misdiagnosed.

- **Epidermoid Cyst**: Usually adherent to the skin, this benign cyst might have a lipomatous feel to it.

- **Neurofibroma**: A benign tumor of the nerve sheath that resembles a lipoma and may manifest as a soft, moveable mass.

CHAPTER 9

PROSPECTS FOR THE FUTURE

Progress in Lipoma Study

Genetic Insights: New investigations into the genetics of lipomas have revealed particular genetic alterations linked to the growth of these tumors.

- **Molecular Pathways:** Targeted medicines have been made possible by gaining an understanding of the molecular pathways underlying lipoma growth.

- **Immunotherapy:** Investigating immunotherapeutic methods of treating lipomas, which make use of the immune system to specifically target and eradicate lipoma cells.

Research on Stem Cells: Examining how stem cells contribute to the development of lipomas and possible regenerative treatments.

New Technologies in the Diagnosis of Lipomatosis

- **MRI Imaging:** Improvements in MRI technology have increased the precision of lipoma identification and diagnosis.

- **CT and Ultrasound Scans:** Making use of CT and Ultrasound scans to precisely locate and evaluate lipomas.

- **Biopsy Methodologies:** Advancements in minimally invasive biopsy methods for conclusive lipoma identification.

- **Digital Pathology:** Using digital pathology instruments to analyze lipomas more quickly and precisely.

Customised Medicine and Treatment for Lipomatosis

- **Genomic Profiling:** Adapting therapy to the lipoma's genetic profile to maximize effectiveness.

Targeted Therapies: Creating medications that target the precise molecular pathways that fuel the growth of lipomas.

Patient-Specific Approaches: Developing individualized treatment regimens by taking into account each patient's unique characteristics, including age, health, and lipoma location.

- **Combination Therapies:** Investigating how combining various therapy modalities can have a synergistic effect for the best results.

Possible Treatments for Lipomas

Gene Editing: Examining whether genetic defects underlying lipomas may be corrected by gene editing techniques such as CRISPR/Cas9.

- **Regenerative Medicine:** Investigating regenerative methods to substitute healthy tissue with lipoma tissue.

Immunotherapy: Using the immune system to eradicate lipoma cells.

Nanomedicine: Targeted delivery of therapeutic medicines to lipomas via nanoparticles.

Ethical Issues in Research on Lipomas

- **Informed Consent:** Making sure patients are completely aware of the advantages and disadvantages of taking part in lipoma research.

- **Privacy and Confidentiality:** Preserving patient information and keeping it private at all times when conducting research.

- **Equitable Access:** Dealing with problems related to varied communities' access to clinical trials and cutting-edge treatments.

- **Patient Autonomy:** Upholding patients' freedom to choose wisely whether or not to participate in research trials.

Lipoma's Global Impact

Economic Burden: Evaluating the financial burden that lipoma management places on international healthcare systems.

- **Quality of Life:** Recognising how lipomas affect patients' quality of life on a physical and psychological level.

- **Assignment of Resources:** Juggling resources for lipoma treatment with other medical needs.

- **International Collaboration:** Promoting cooperation amongst nations to exchange best practices and advance lipoma research more quickly.

Awareness Campaigns for Lipomas

- **Education and Information:** Educating medical professionals and the general public about lipomas, their diagnosis, and available treatments.

- **Support Networks:** Creating networks and resources to assist people with lipomas and those who care for them.

- **Community Engagement:** Bringing up topics related to lipoma awareness, prevention, and early identification in local communities.

- **Advocacy Initiatives:** Pushing for more financing and support for studies about lipomas.

Lipoma Patient Advocacy

Giving patients information about lipomas and their treatment alternatives will empower them.

- **Advocacy Groups:** To strengthen patient voices and promote good change, supporting and working in tandem with patient advocacy groups.

- **Policy Influence:** Promoting laws that increase lipoma sufferers' access to high-quality medical care and treatment alternatives.

- **Research Participation:** Promoting patient involvement in investigations and clinical trials to further the understanding of lipoma.

AI's Function in Lipoma Management

- **Diagnostic Support:** Artificial intelligence algorithms support precise and effective lipoma diagnosis using imaging data.

- **Treatment Planning:** AI-powered instruments supporting medical professionals in creating customized treatment regimens based on patient information and research findings.

- **Data Analysis:** Making use of AI to examine huge datasets to spot trends and patterns in the emergence and spread of lipomas.

Predictive Modelling: Using AI models to forecast how lipoma patients would react to various treatment modalities and their prognosis.

Public Health and Lipoma Initiatives

Preventive Measures: Informing people about lifestyle choices and practices that may be linked to the development of lipomas.

- **Screening Programmes:** Starting screening initiatives will help identify lipomas early on, particularly in high-risk groups.

Healthcare Infrastructure: Enhancing the system of healthcare to guarantee prompt diagnosis and treatment of lipomas.

- **Research Funding:** Fighting for financing from the public health system to promote research on lipomas and novel treatment approaches.

CHAPTER 10

COMPREHENDING LIPOMA'S ANATOMY

Lipoma Structure

Benign tumors called lipomas are made of adipose tissue or fat tissue. They are usually enclosed in a fibrous capsule and have a soft, rubbery touch. Their encapsulation sets them apart from other growths connected to fat, such as lipomatosis, which is ill-defined.

Material Constituency

Mature adipocytes, specialized fat cells that store energy as fat, are the primary biological constituent of lipomas. The majority of the tumor is composed of these cells, which are often all the same size and shape.

Hereditary Elements

There is evidence pointing to a genetic propensity for lipomas, even if the actual etiology of the condition is still unknown. Multiple lipomas are more likely to occur in people with specific genetic disorders, such as familial multiple lipomatosis.

Differences Between Other Tumours and Lipoma

The main way that lipomas are different from other tumors is in the makeup of their cells. Different types of cells can be seen in tumors other than lipomas, like muscle cells in myolipomas or blood vessel cells in angiolipomas.

Adipocytes' Part in the Formation of Lipomas

Adipocytes multiply and aggregate within the fibrous capsule, gradually generating the tumor's distinctive soft mass, which is a key factor in the creation of lipomas.

Effect on Adjacent Tissues

Lipomas typically don't aggressively invade neighboring tissues and are non-invasive. They may, however, enlarge to the point that they put pressure on surrounding structures, resulting in symptoms like pain or limited mobility.

Patterns of Lipomato Growth

Lipomas frequently go years without showing any symptoms. They can grow slowly over time. Individual differences may exist in the pace of growth, and certain lipomas may exhibit stable growth or even spontaneous regression.

Features, Both Microscopic and Macroscopic

Under the microscope, lipomas have a homogeneous appearance with mature adipocytes grouped into lobules and divided by fibrous septae. Because of their high-fat content, they appear macroscopic as soft, well-circumscribed aggregates with a yellowish tint.

Investigation Histopathological

Using a microscope, tissue samples from the lipoma are examined histopathologically. By confirming the existence of mature adipocytes and ruling out any malignant characteristics, this examination aids in distinguishing lipomas from more worrisome tumors.

Aspects of Radiography

Because of their fatty content, lipomas usually present as well-defined, homogenous masses on imaging examinations such as ultrasonography, CT scans, or MRI with low density on CT scans and high signal intensity on MRI. These features help distinguish them from other soft tissue tumors and aid in diagnosis.